Cure Arthritis Naturally

Get Rid of Your Pain Forever

By Kelly Timber

Table of Contents

INTRODUCTION

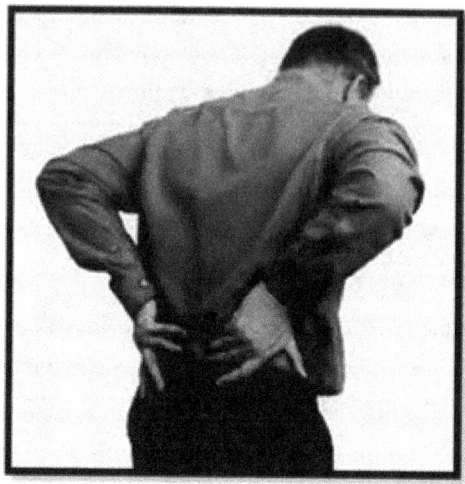

Arthritis cannot be termed as a single disease and it covers more than 100 medical problems. It is more like a generic term that is used for ailments that causes stiffness, pain or swelling. The cartilage within the joints may face a disruption due to arthritis pain.

In this book, we will provide you a strong foundation on what is arthritis and how to reverse arthritis naturally. We will get into the details about what exactly arthritis is as well as what the different forms of arthritis people can suffer from. We will talk about the different treatment options that are available as well as the pros and cons that comes with this ailment. It is our hope that after reading this book you will have a better understanding of this disease and can help yourself as well as others to deal with this condition.

WE ARE NOT DOCTORS NOR DO WE PERSONALLY ENDORSE ANYTHING THAT IS WRITTEN IN THIS BOOK. THIS IS FOR EDUCATION PURPOSES ONLY.

WHAT IS ARTHRITIS

Arthritis is derived from Greek word "Arthron" meaning joint and Latin word "itis" means inflammation.

Arthritis is a kind of joint disorder, which is caused due to the tenderness of one or more joints in the human body. When you say the word "Arthritis", you are covering a condition that includes pain, inflation, stiffness and not a specific form of the disease.

There are over 100 different forms of Arthritis, of which the most common is Osteoarthritis. Osteoarthritis can occur due to a number of factors. It is mostly caused because of trauma in the joints due to accidents or if a person is hit directly on the joint by some hard material. You may also get osteoarthritis, if you suffer from any form of disease that affects the bones and tissues of the body. It is also most common among elderly people.

The major complaint or symptoms of arthritis are joint pain. A person suffering from arthritis feels a constant pain on his or her joints, ligaments, tendons or bursas. The pain is caused by inflammation in the joints. Inflammation is generally the result of wear and tear on the body, muscle strain or any disease in the course of a lifetime.

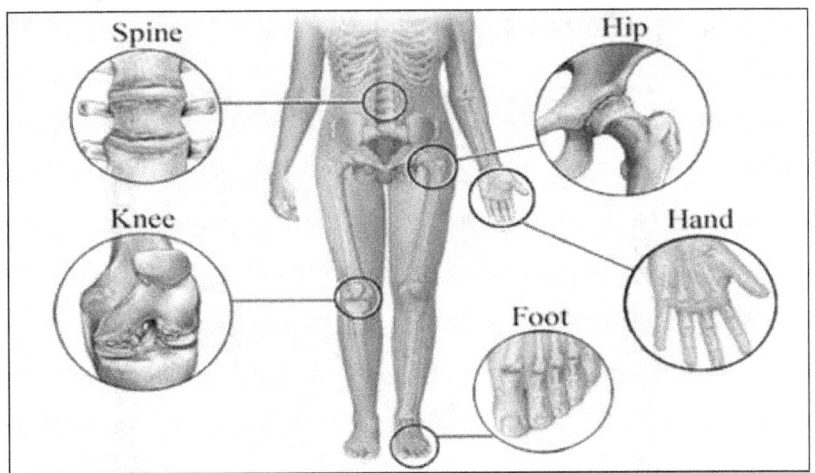

Listed below are the most common forms of arthritis and the conditions they inherit.

OSTEOARTHRITIS

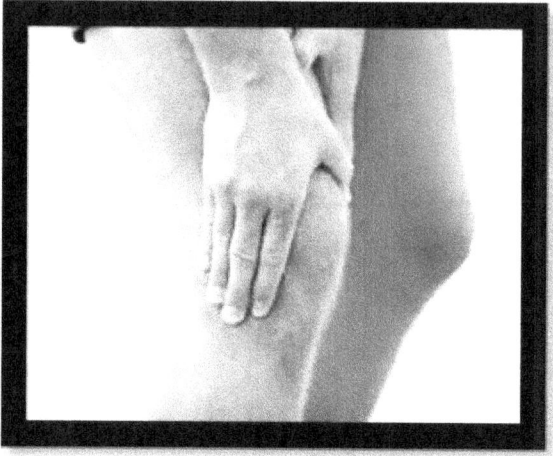

Osteoarthritis is known as the degenerative form of arthritis. It mainly affects the cartilages of the joints, which are a type of tissue that covers the end part of the bones. In osteoarthritis, the above layer of cartilages wear away and gradually breaks down. Due to this wearing away of the cartilages, the bones starts rubbing together, which causes swelling and pain. Osteoarthritis can be heredity, or may be caused due to developmental or metabolic issues.

Cartilage is the firm, rubbery tissue that cushions your bones at the joints and allows the bones to glide over one another. If the cartilage breaks down and wears away, the bones rub together. This may cause pain, swelling and stiffness.

Treatment generally involves a combination of exercise, lifestyle modification and diet. The disease often becomes debilitating and joint replacement surgery may be required to improve the quality of life.

The main symptom of osteoarthritis is joint pain, which causes the loss of mobility and often results in sustained stiffness in the joints. This kind of pain is generally felt as a sharp burning sensation in the associated muscles and tendons. Osteoarthritis can cause a cracking noise when the affected joint is moved or touched. People may experience muscle spasms and contractions in the affected areas. Occasionally, the joint may also be filled with fluid. Some people report increased pain associated with cold temperature, high humidity, and/or a dropping of paramedic pressure.

Osteoarthritis or OA may run in families. Other conditions such as being overweight increases the risk of OA in the hip area, knees, ankles and foot joints because the extra weight in a human body causes more wear and tear.

Fractures or other joint injuries can lead to OA at a later phase in life. This includes cartilage and ligament injuries in the joints. Any type of movement that involve kneeling or squatting for more than an hour a day puts you at the highest risk of OA. Jobs that involve lifting, climbing stairs and walking may also lead to this ailment.

Those who play sports that involve direct impact on the joint such as football, twisting such as basketball, soccer or simply throwing also increases the risk of arthritis.

Medical conditions that can lead to OA may include but are not limited to:

1. Bleeding disorders like bleeding in the joint such as hemophilia.

2. Disorders that block the blood supply to a joint and leads to vascular necrosis.

3. Other forms of arthritis

RHEUMATOID ARTHRITIS

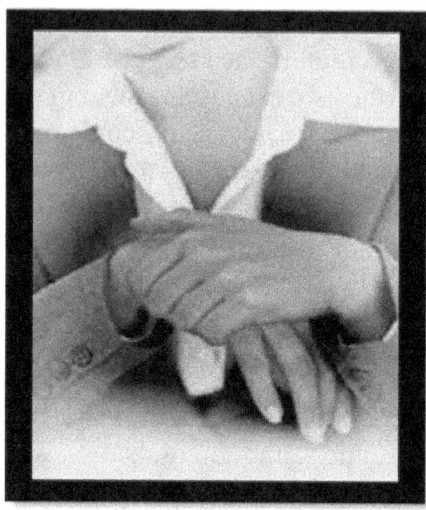

Rheumatoid arthritis or RA is a form of autoimmune disease that may disturb the pulmonary and systemic circulation of blood and may affect many organs and tissues by attacking the flexible joints of the hands and feet. This form of arthritis can lead to a painful or disabling condition, which can cause subsequent declines in functionality and mobility of the entire body, if it is not adequately treated at the right time.

The cause of RA is unknown, but as it is a form of autoimmune disease, where the immune system mistakenly starts attacking the tissue or cells of human body.

RA can happen at any time of life but is more common amongst middle-age women. Even though there is no exact known cause for this condition, researchers suspect that infection, genes and hormonal changes may be linked to this form of arthritis.

RA usually affects joints both the sides of the body correspondingly. Fingers, wrists, feet, knees and ankles are areas that are most commonly affected by this form of arthritis. The disease often contracts slowly and affects the body over several years. The onset of this disease occurs with mild joint pain, stiffness and fatigue.

Joint symptoms may include but are not limited to the following:

Morning stiffness may last for at least one hour. Joint pain is often felt on the same joint on both sides of the body and over a period of time the joints may lose their range of motion, which may also result in slight to major deformities in the body.

In severe cases of RA, some people may also experience severe chest pain while taking deep breaths, dry eyes and mouth, burning eyes, itching and abnormal serum discharge. Rheumatoid nodules may begin to form under the skin. People suffering from RA also report of having numbness, itching or burring in the hands and feet as well as face sleep disturbances due to pain.

GOUT AND PSEUDO-GOUT

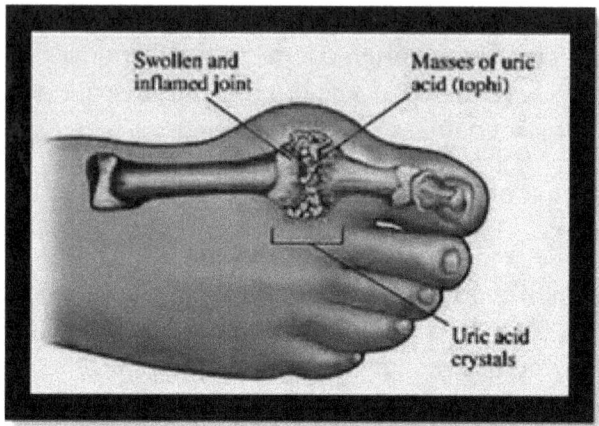

Gout is a form of arthritis. It occurs when uric acid level increases in the blood and causes inflammation in the joints. Acute gout is a painful condition that often affects only one joint in the body. Chronic gout may lead to repeated episodes of pain and inflammation in various joint of the body. Chronic Gout usually affects more than one joint of the body.

Gout increases normal levels of uric acid in the body and this may be caused under the following conditions:

Your body starts generation more uric acid than required at one time and it becomes tough to get rid of the extra level of uric acid. If too much uric acid builds up in the fluid around the joints, the acid begins to form crystals in the body. These crystals will cause the joints to swell or become inflated. This results in pain in the joints.

Like Rheumatoid arthritis, the exact of gout is not known properly. Unlike Rheumatoid arthritis, which mainly targets women, gout is more prevalent in men. Gout may affect women who have attained the age of menopause and as well as people who consume alcohol.

Gout symptoms include but not limited to the following:

It may at times only affect one joint. These are limited to the big toe, knee or ankle joints. Pain related to gout generally starts suddenly and often during night. Pain is often described as throbbing, crushing or excruciating in intensity.

Joints appear warm and red as well as very tender and swollen. Patients suffering from gout may also begin to spike fever. After an attack of gout, it may take a few days before the symptoms to complete disappear. If gout does occur again in future, it may last longer and become more intense than the previous time.

SEPTIC ARTHRITIS

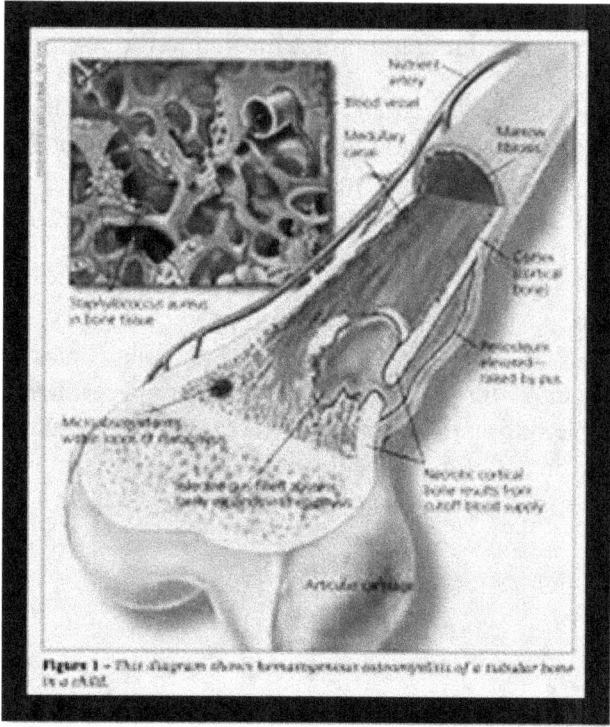

Figure 1 – This diagram shows tenosynovial osteomyelitis of a tubular bone in a child.

Septic arthritis is also known as, "rich man disease". Septic arthritis is caused by one or more microorganisms, which attack the joints of the body. Generally, the joint is smoothened with the supply of fluid, which is better known as joint fluid or synovial fluid.

The normal fluid, which is also sterile, and in case it needs to be cultivated, cultured or even removed in a laboratory, there will be no traces of microorganisms in it. Microorganisms like bacteria, are detectable in the case of septic arthritis.

Similar to gout, usually a single joint is affected in Septic Arthritis, but at times more than one joint is affected. The joints that are affected by the microorganisms, which cause infections, may at times differ.

Bacteria, fungi and various other viruses may be the main cause of septic arthritis. The most typical element of septic arthritis is bacterial infections such as haemophilus influenza and staphylococcus aureus.

In some people, who are mostly endovenous drug abusers and the elderly people, septic arthritis can be caused by Pseudomonas spp. and E. coli. Neisseria gonorrhea is very common in sexually dynamic young people and salmonella app is found in small children and among people suffering from sickle cell disease. Bacteria such Mycobacterium tuberculosis and spirochete bacterium can be causes of septic arthritis and Lyme disease.

Septic arthritis can be caused by viruses such as mumps, hepatitis A, B, C, Herpes virus, parvovirus B19, HIV (AIDS virus) HTLV-1, coxsackle viruses, adenovirus and Ebola. Similar to virus, fungus such as coccidiomyces, histoplasma and blastomyces can also be a cause of septic arthritis.

ANKLOSING SPONDYLITIS

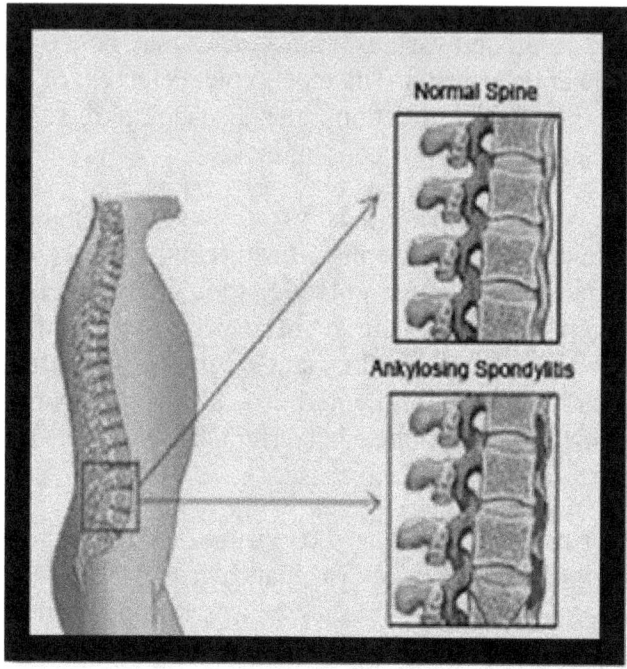

Ankylosing Spondylitis is a form of arthritis that can have long-term consequences. It affects the bones and joints at the base of the spine where it connects to the pelvis. These joints become swollen and inflamed. This may lead the spinal bones to join or fuse.

The cause of Ankylosing Spondylitis is unknown. Genes seem to play a role in its development. The disease most often begins between the ages of 20 and 40, but in exceptional cases, it may occur as a young age of 10. This form of arthritis appears to affect more males than females.

The disease starts with low back pain that comes and goes. Low back pain starts increasing as the disease starts to progress in the human body. Pain and stiffness are worse during the morning time, at night, and when you are less active. The best way to start to alleviate the pain is to start moving around, exercising or just maintain an active and healthy lifestyle.

Back pain may begin in the sacroiliac joints between the pelvis and spine. Over a period, this condition may affect the entire spine. People suffering from this form of arthritis may lose flexibility in their lower spine. The condition may affect the joints between your ribs, causing breathing problems due to lack of expanding the chest properly.

Treatment for this form of arthritis may include a prescription from your doctor for anti-inflammatory drugs to reduce swelling and pain. Surgery may be done if pain or joint damage is severe.

JUVENILE IDIOPATHIC ARTHRITIS

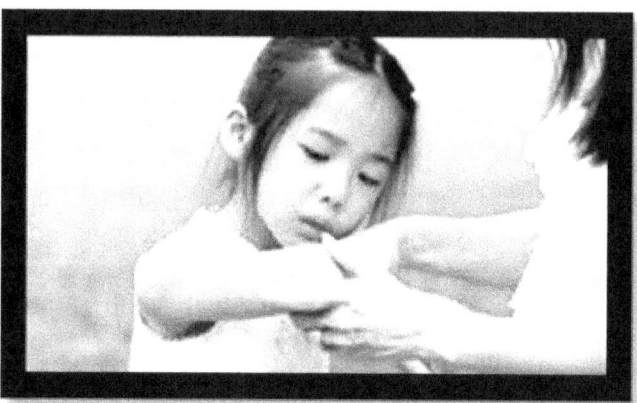

Juvenile Arthritis or JA refers to the form of arthritis or arthritis-related condition that develops in children or teenagers who are less than 18 years of age.

There are currently over 249,000 children under the age of 18 who are victim of this disease worldwide.

Common symptoms of juvenile arthritis include pain, swelling, tenderness and stiffness of joints causing limited motion. Joint contracture results from a painful joint in a flexed position for extended period. This condition may lead to damage of joint cartilage, joint deformation and impaired use of the joint, altered growth of bone and joints that may lead to a short stature of the person.

Types of Juvenile Arthritis include JRA, also known as Polyarticular juvenile rheumatoid arthritis and JIA, also known as Juvenile idiopathic arthritis. Girls are more affected by this form of arthritis than boys are. This form of arthritis more commonly affects the wrists, knees and ankles. It often affects a joint on one side of the body, mostly the knees.

The cure of juvenile arthritis may vary considering the form of the ailment. The primary goal of treating JA is by keeping a check on any form of swelling, preventing joint damage, controlling inflammation and at the same time maximizing the body functional abilities.

Small children can be treated in various ways like physical activity, physical or occupational therapy, medication, health education, dental as well as eye care and proper nutrition.

STILLS DISEASE

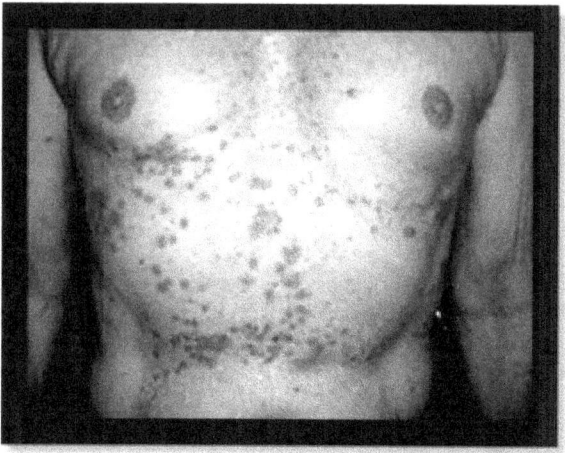

Adult onset stills disease is a systemic and pulmonary disease. Stills disease is commonly associated with a high spiking fever and a rash that does not cause any itching. With stills disease, you will always have a joint pain and inflammation. The cause for stills disease, like most other form of arthritis we have discussed, is unknown. Stills disease can lead to inflammation of internal organs. Classic blood tests that are done for rheumatic diseases that show negative result in this disease. Treatment is directed towards the individual areas of inflammation.

Stills disease can cause serious damage to the joints, particularly the writs. It can also impair the function of the heart and lungs. Treatments of stills disease is directed towards the individual areas of inflammation. Anti-inflammatory drugs such as aspirin often control many symptoms of this disease.

Now that we know about arthritis and its different forms, let us know about the cures and treatments related to the disease. Before you decide to start any treatment for your condition, make sure you consult a doctor or physician before taking anything that was not prescribed to you. Make sure that not anything that you do or try will affect any other condition that you may have. Your health and safety should be your main concern.

TREATMENTS, REMEDIES AND MORE

Ever since the beginning of time, people have been dealing with arthritis. People have been doing everything from spiritual healing to designer drugs to curb the pain, arthritis causes. They are trying to do anything and everything that they can think of to alleviate the pain.

Even though there has been great advancements in medical research there is no cure for this disease in most cases. The main question comes into play is, if you are going to try prescription drugs, natural herbs, diet and exercise, surgery or some combination of treatments.

Listed in the following pages are options that you may try.

Herbs

Herbs are an essential part of our diet. In the following section, I will give you some herbs that have been known to relief the arthritis pain and other ailments as well. Please consult your doctor before taking any herbs for curbing arthritis pain.

Alfalfa

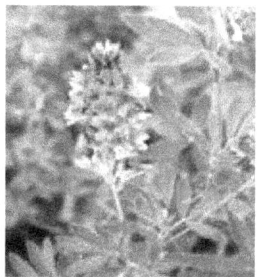

Supplements from natural alfalfa possess quite a number of assets that helps in successfully softening uric acid that may cause gout. This will help it to successfully pass through your kidneys. Alfalfa is better known as the "The father of all foods" and it mostly contains a depot of nutrients and minerals, which is essential in combating the symptoms of arthritis.

Alfalfa does not have any side effects and people who use it have never complained of any problem due to its use. But, always follow the dosage that has been prescribed to you. There has been no study regarding any intercommunication of traditional pharmaceuticals and alfalfa.

Boswellia

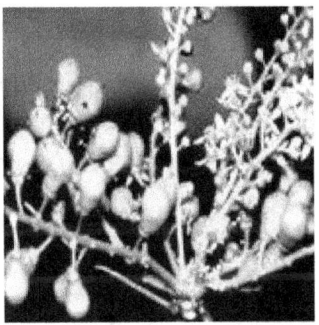

Boswellia is a tree found in India known for its gum resin, which has many pharmacological uses, particularly as an anti-inflammatory. It is also known as Indian Frankincense, salaiguggal and boswellin. Its proper botanic name is boswelliaserraia. Boswellia has been used for thousands of years to treat many types of medical conditions.

Cat's Claw

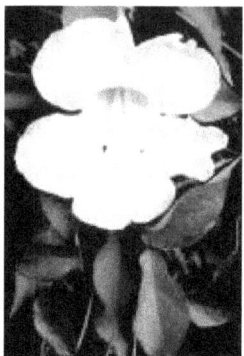

Cat's claw is a plant, which is primarily used for medicinal purpose. There are two separate species of cat's claw. The first is Uncariatomentosa and the other is Uncariaguianensis. Uncariatomentosa is most commonly used in the United States while UncariaGuianensis is more commonly found in Europe.

Cat's claw can help with various digestive disorders including swelling and pain of the large intestine. Inflammation of the lower bowels, inflammation of the inner stomach, stomach ulcers, hemorrhoids and leaky bowl syndrome.

It has also been known that people during ancient times have used Cat's Claw for viral infections, including shingles, cold sores and aids. Cat's claw is also good in easing the symptoms of rheumatoid arthritis. When you are looking for a plant that has a lot of uses, cat's claw is always considered. However, check with your doctor before taking any type of drug with Cat's claw as one of the ingredients.

Ginger

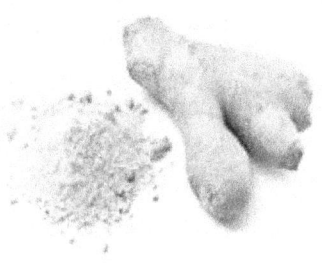

Fragrant herbs and spices such as ginger, is one of the most powerful weapons, which helps in combating inflammation from a natural perspective. Inflammation causes and contributes to obesity, diabetes, cardiovascular disease, Alzheimer's disease and many types of cancer.

Ginger contains dozens powerful and potent inflammation-fighting substances such as phytonutrients, which is also called gingerls. Gingerls attack the inflammation caused by arthritis causing the swelling to subside alleviating the pain.

Cayenne Peppers

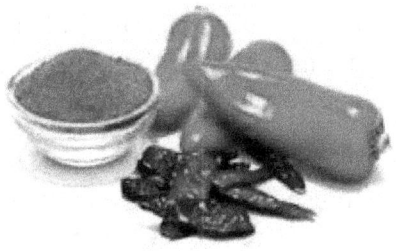

Cayenne peppers contain an ingredient known as capsaicin that helps in relieving the pain. This is done by inhibiting the release of substance P, which is a neurotransmitter responsible for transmitting pain sensations.

Pain characterizes all forms of arthritis, including osteoarthritis, rheumatoid arthritis and gout. Capsaicin in cayenne has potent pain-relieving effects. When applied in cream or ointment form, capsaicin initially causes a brief stinging sensation, which stimulates the pain nerves. It then gradually reduces substance P, a chemical necessary for nerves to send pain signals.

Nettle Leaf

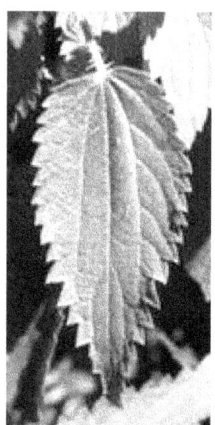

Nettle leaf is a good source of medicine to curb arthritis pain. Stinging nettle as it is generally called is used in many ways to cure ailments such as enlarged prostate, night-time urination and other leading related to the urinary track system.

Many people also use nettle leaf to cure their aches and pains. Nevertheless, there is not enough scientific evidence to determine whether it is effective for the previously mentioned problems.

Noni

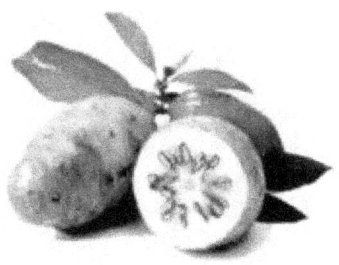

Noni is known as the "Sacred Plant" to the Polynesian people in the south Pacific. It has been used for more than 2,000 years for pain, arthritis and other health problems. Using the plant as a drink can be used to cure arthritis due to its anti-inflammatory effects.

Olive Leaf Extract

Olive is a tree and people use oil from the olive fruits and seeds such as water extracts of the fruit and the leaves to make medicine. Olive oil is used to prevent heart attacks, strokes, breast cancer, colorectal cancer, rheumatoid arthritis and migraine headaches.

Some people use the olive oil to treat constipation, high cholesterol, high blood pressure, blood pressure problems and much more. Olive oil has a wide range of uses and should be added to your daily diet.

Turmeric

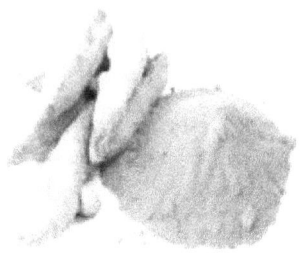

Turmeric contains curcumin, which has anti-inflammatory and pain relieving properties. It is good for inflammatory conditions such as arthritis.

Turmeric is a rhizomatous herbaceous plant of the ginger family. It is native to tropical Indian subcontinent and needs temperatures between 20 and 30 degrees Celsius to grow and thrive.

Willow Bark

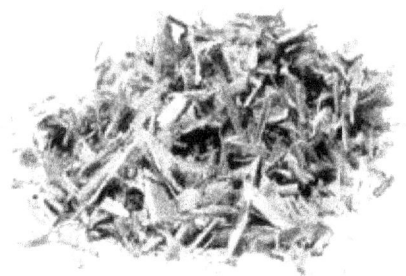

The bark of the Willow tree is known as the Willow bark and it has a wide range of varieties like European Willow, White Willow, Pussy Willow, Black Willow, Crack Willow and the Purple Willow. The bark is used to make several types of medicines.

The bark from the willow tree acts on the body similar to aspirin. Besides being able to help with rheumatoid arthritis, osteoarthritis pain and gout, willow bark can assist in curbing muscle pain, headaches, menstrual cramps and a disease of the spine called ankylosing spondylitis.

Borage Seed Oil

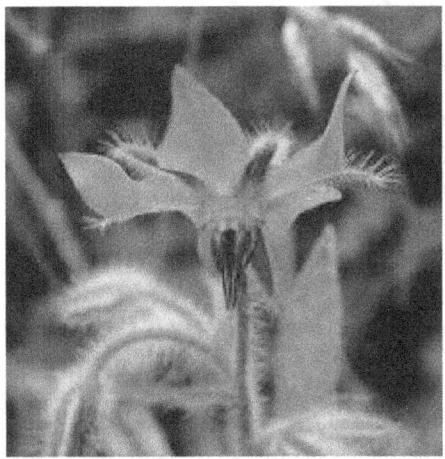

Borage seed oil has the highest amount of y-linolenic acid (GLA) of seed oils. Taking a dosage of 1800 milligrams a day may be effective in pain control but fish oil has a better mixture of fatty acids to reduce TNF and COX-2

Brigham Tea

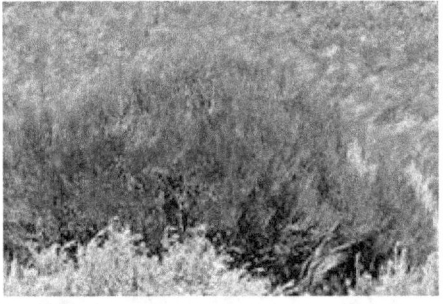

The herbal acids found in Brigham tea helps to curb pain in many parts of the body. The acids help in eliminating toxic substances in the bowels. It is also a great healer for arthritis. You can either consume the tea as a drink or you can crush up the leaves and rub the oils onto your joints to help alleviate the symptoms of arthritis.

Buchu Leaves

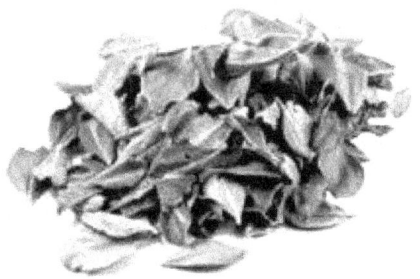

The Buchu leaves also acts as a good pain reliever. The plant's leaf are used to make a medicine that helps with several forms of arthritis as well as urinary tract infection and bladder infections. It also helps to flush out the kidneys and assist in treating sexually transmitted diseases.

Burdock Root

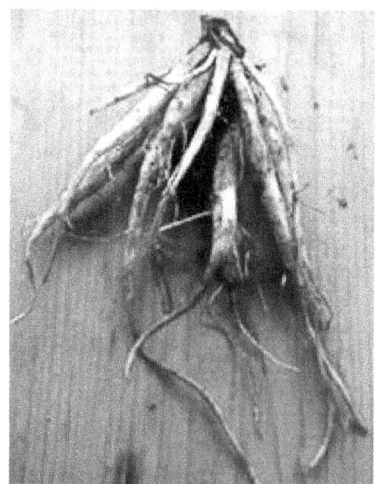

Burdock Root is also known as Fox Coat, Beggars Buttons and Great Bur. It is a broad-leaved perennial herb with spiny, thistle-like flowers. The Burdock Root plant found in native North America, Africa and Western Europe.

Burdock Root contains a wide range of useful chemicals like copper, biotin, manganese, vitamins B and E, iron, sulfur, Zinc and inulin. The part of the Burdock root that tastes sweet and leaves is used for medicinal purposes.

To prepare a Burdock tea, you will need to boil 4 cups of fresh water. Finely chop 2 tablespoons of fresh Burdock Root. If you do not have fresh root available you may use 2 teaspoons of dried root as an alternative.

Add the root to the boiling water and allow to simmer for 10 minutes. Then turn off the flame and strain the mixture. Sip slowly while it is warm.

Drink 3-4 cups daily for getting rid of arthritis pain.

Celery Seed

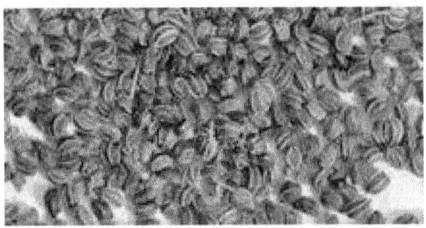

Celery seeds are an effective anti-inflammatory to reduce arthritis symptoms. Traditionally, ancient medical practice in India used celery seed for rheumatoid symptoms. Modern research has identified many phenolic and flavonoid antioxidants with anti-inflammatory potential in celery seed.

Celery seeds can be found in many anti-inflammatory medications. Most of these medicines can be purchased over the counter.

Corn Silk

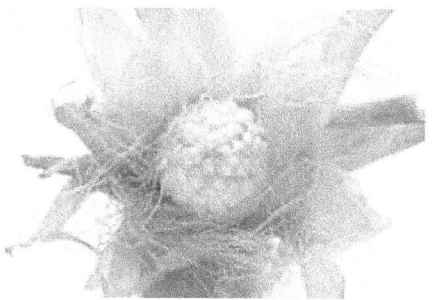

Corn silk is not only used in lessening the symptoms of arthritis, it can also help with bladder infections, inflammation of the urinary system, inflammation of the prostate, kidney stones and also help to curb the bed-wetting problems in children.

It can also be used to treat congestive heart failure, diabetes, high blood pressure, fatigue and high cholesterol.

Corn silk contains proteins, carbohydrates, vitamins, minerals and fiber. They also contain chemicals that may act like a water pill or more commonly known as a diuretics.

Devils Claw

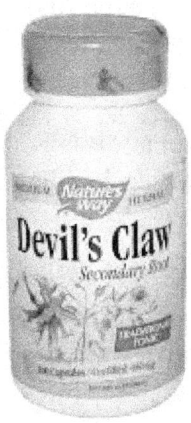

In Germany, Devil's Claw is widely used for arthritis pain in the back, knee and hip.

Devils Claw is a desert plant that grows in southern Africa and is named for the miniature claw-like hooks that cover its fruit. For centuries, the root was dried and chopped to be used as remedies to treat pain and indigestion. It was also used to treat soars and other skin problems.

In recent years, scientists have studied its effects on arthritis that is located mainly in the knee and hip. The results have been promising and those who have been using Devil's Claw swear by its results.

Parsley Tea

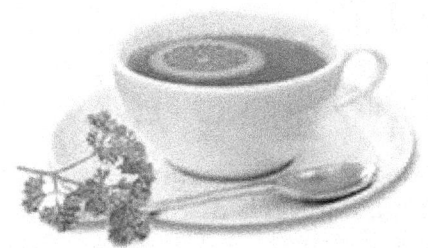

When you think of parsley the first thing that comes to mind is the little green thing they is put on the side of your plate in fancy restaurants that is eventually discarded.

Parsley is an amazing plant. It is beneficial as a digestive aid, detoxifier and cleanser. Parsley can also help in making you smell better.

Parsley has a variety of nutrients that may protect us against various forms of cancer. It is rich in antioxidants like vitamin C and beta carotene. Parsley also contains some lesser known flavonoids like apigenin, luteolin and chrysoeriol.

Yucca

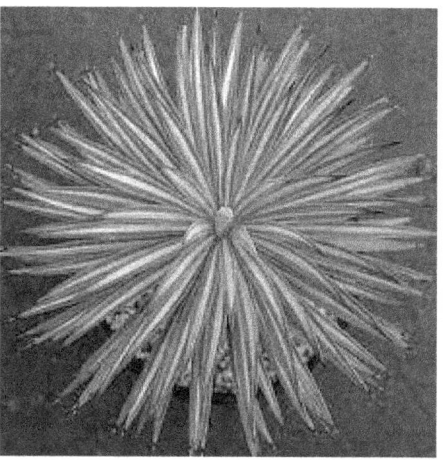

The spiny Yucca plant, which has been used for centuries as a staple food for the Indians of south-western United States, may offer some hope for millions of people who suffer from arthritis.

How this amazing plant aids in arthritis is not exactly known. A study in California discovered that those who took the Yucca compound in pill form experienced dramatic alleviation of pain in areas they were affected by arthritis. More studies are needed to be conducted before this plant can become a mainstream option but it also has additional qualities of possible treatments, which are still to be discovered.

In the next section of the book we will be discussing diet factors. We will tell you what types of food that you can eat and what food you should avoid and why.

DIET FACTORS

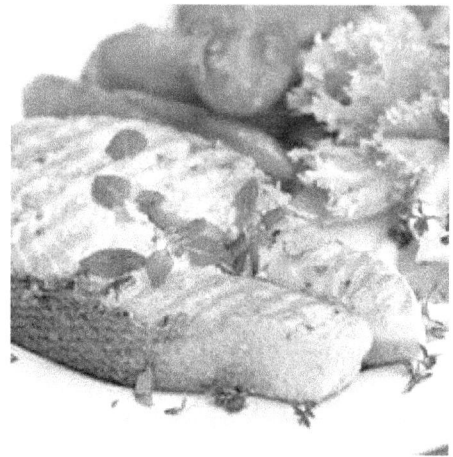

It is commonly said, "you are what you eat". This is true in the sense that you food is absorbed by the body, which is then used to aid in our growth and development. As we age, we require to change our diet to fit our body's changing needs. When we were younger, we were able to eat practically anything that we wanted to and not gain weight or affect our bodies to a considerable degree.

However, as we get older our food habits change. We are required to take in different nutrients to keep our bones and muscles healthy. In this chapter, we will give you a better understanding of what you should and shouldn't eat and why.

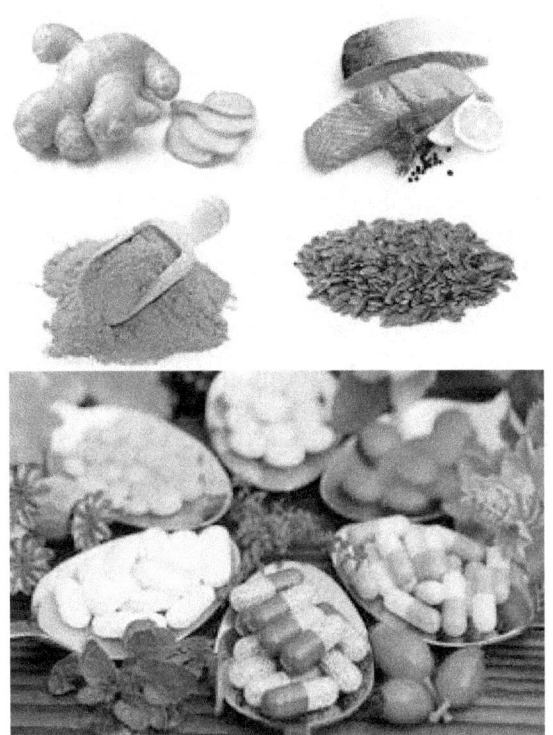

WHAT TO EAT

If you have arthritis, it is highly recommended that you eat food items that are high in sulfer content. I know what you are thinking. "Sulfer?" Isn't sulfer smell like rotten eggs? Well, yes! It does. It is also the most plentiful mineral in your body.

The sulfer mineral can be found in your nerve cells, connective tissues, skin, nails and hair. Sulfer is also known to support cardiac health and liver function and has the potential to assist in curbing various forms of cancer. Since, sulfer is so abundant in our bodies there has been no dietary recommendations placed on it.

Asparagus

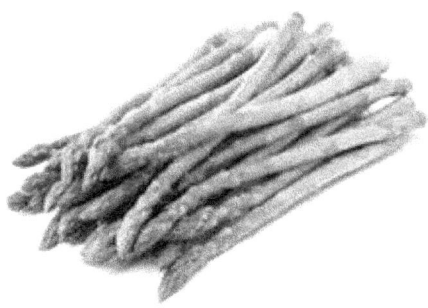

Asparagus is one of the most nutritionally well-balanced vegetable that nature provides. Asparagus is the leading supplier of folic acid among all the vegetables that we eat. Folic acid is responsible for blood cell formation, growth and prevention of liver disease.

Asparagus is low in calories, only 20 per 5.3 oz serving. It contains no fat or cholesterol. It is very low in sodium and is also a good source of potassium. For those who need fiber in their diet it also contains 3 grams per serving. Asparagus also contains folacin, thiamin, vitamin B6. With those who have arthritis and other ailments, it can be great diet for them.

Brocoli

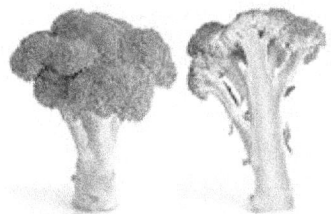

Brocoli is a curciferous vegetable that is stuffed with vitamins, A, B, K, C as well as nutrients such as potassium, zinc and fiber. Broccoli also contain sulfer, which is great for those who suffer with arthritis.

Cabbage

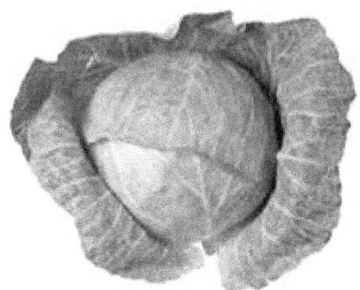

Cabbage is another great vegetable that you can help in getting rid of arthritis pain. Unlike some vegetables, that you eat to gain its benefits, cabbage can be used externally to gain relief from arthritis pain.

Here are the steps you need to remember to get the external benefits of cabbage:

Step 1: Place cabbage leaves, preferably from red cabbage on a cutting board and cut off the hard stem with a sharp knife. Then use a wine bottle, rolling pin or meat hammer to gently bruise the leaves releasing some of the cabbage juices.

Step 2: Wrap the cabbage leaves in foil and place in the oven for a few minutes to warm them. This will make the leaves pliable. Make sure that the leaves are warm. Don't cook or over heat them.

Step 3: Wrap the warm cabbage leaves around the painful joint until it is completely encased with the leaves. If leaves are too hot, allow them to cool for a minute before applying on the skin. Hold the leaves and wrap with a self-stick gauze bandage covering the entire mass with plastic wrap or aluminum foil to hold the warm feeling.

Step 4: Leave the cabbage leaves wrapped around your joint for at least an hour if not longer. Repeat this process using new cabbage leaves on a daily basis for continued relief.

STEP 5: When you have completed this process, unwrap the cabbage leaves and discard them.

Cauliflower

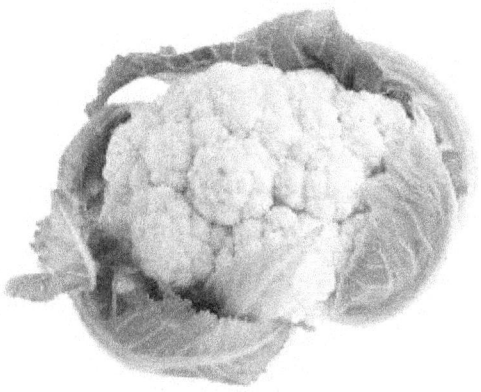

Cauliflower is the only vegetable that has been proven to cure Rheumatoid arthritis. Studies have shown that eating 4 to 7 servings a week helps in having strong joints. Eating cauliflower also aids in the easing of gout symptoms.

Chives

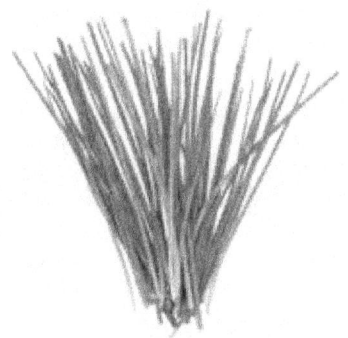

Chives are a great addition to your diet. The juice from the chives plant can be applied to areas in the body that is affected by arthritis. This will help in getting rid of the pain. Chives are also good for the kidneys, liver and stomach. Chives can also be consumed when you have injuries as they aid in the release of swelling and promote healing.

Eggs

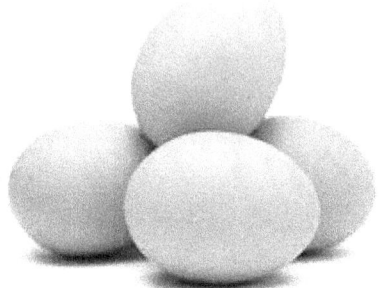

Eatting eggs is a great way to help curb arthritis pain. Eggs contain sulfer, which aids in the body's healing process. If you are allergic to eggs you must consult your doctor or look at the other options that are available for arthritis pain relief.

Fish

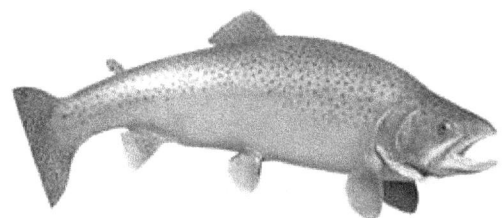

Eatting one portion of oily fish per week will aid you in the reduction of rheumatoid arthritis. The oil in fish helps in giving relief to arthritis pain.

Garlic

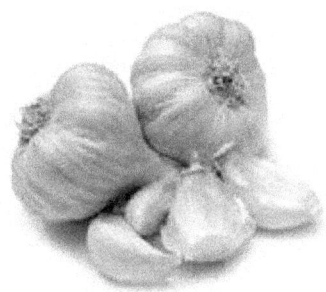

Garlic is a wonderful item, which can be added to your diet. It helps in curing rheumatoid arthritis as well as various other ailments. Garlic can reduce pain and inflamation. Garlic inhibits the formation of free radicals that can cause joint damage. Garlic is anti-bacterial, anti-viral, anti-fungal and may protect against many forms of cancers as well. Garlic also has cardiovascular benefits. It can reduce blood pressure and cholesterol, which helps to prevent against atherosclerosis. Studies have shown that eating both cooked and raw garlic together provides a better health benefit.

Kale

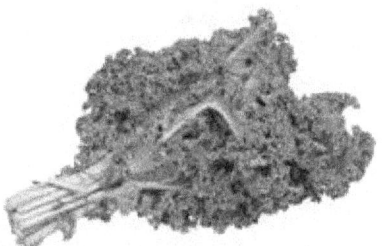

Kale is another great vegetable to eat with arthritis. It contains sulfer as well as other vitamins that aid in the production of pain relief.

Leeks

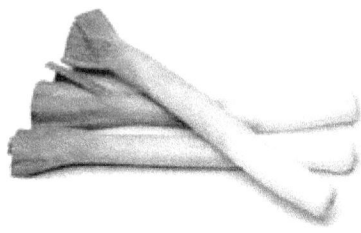

Leeks, like onion and garlic, is another vegetable that aids in the relief of joint pain. It is an anti-inflamintory that helps to soothe inflamation in joints. With their unique combination of flavonoids and sulfur-containing nutrients, eating leeks on a regular basis is a valued addition to your diet.

Very few people know how to cook leeks. It is reccomended that you slice them into thin pieces and prepare them using the saute' method.

Onions

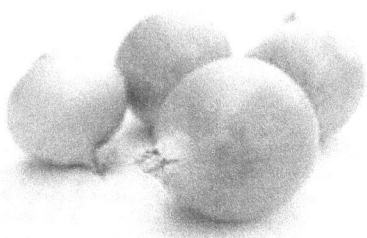

Onions are not just for flavoring your food or to cover in batter at the outback. Onions are low in calories, have virtually no fat and are loaded with healthy components that fight inflamation.

Onions are one of the richest sources of flavonoids. These are the antioxidants that mop up the radicals in your body's cells before they have a chance to cause harm. Onions have also been known to inhibit inflamation causing leukotrienes, prostaglandins and histamines in osteoarthritis and rheumatoid arthritis as well as reduce heart disease and other ailments.

Shallots

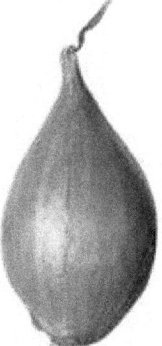

Shallots are from the same family as onions. They have anti-inflamatory qualities. Taken on a regular basis, shallots will help in reducing inflamation for those suffering from arthritis.

Soy Beans

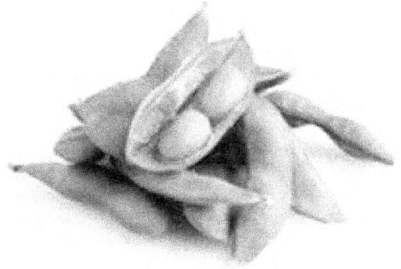

Soybean has been a part of human diet for almost 5000 years. Unlike most plant foods, soy beans are high in protein content. Soy in your diet also lowers cholesterol level, saturates fats and lowers the chance for heart disease. Soy has also been linked to reduce symptoms of menopause and the risk of **osteoporosis**. Soy products are helpful in preventing endometrial cancer, various forms of hormone-dependant cancers including breast cancer and prostate cancer.

CONCLUSION

There is no specific treatment for osteoarthritis or rheumatoid arthritis. The treatment options may differ that depends on the kind of arthritis. One of the most important healing process is physical therapy that include weight control by the means of proper exercise, changes in lifestyle, medications, orthopedic bracing etc.

At times, joint replacement may also be required considering the form of arthritis. Medications can be helpful to curb inflations in joints, which decreases the pain. If the inflation is reduced or checked then they won't cause any further damage.

Natural herbs are also beneficial to curb arthritis as they help in maintaining proper blood supply to the joints. Various types of treatments are used to treat arthritis. Some may have side effects and should be taken as prescribed by the doctor. Hence, it is always good to opt for home-made remedies or natural therapies.

www.ingramcontent.com/pod-product-compliance
Lightning Source LLC
Chambersburg PA
CBHW070840290526
45795CB00002B/929